Sirtfood di
Lo‹

The complete recipe book, lose weight, burn fat and lose weight (includes a step-by-step meal plan with recipes!)

© Copyright 2020 by Mattias Gervy - All rights reserved.

The following Book is reproduced below with the goal of providing information that is as accurate and reliable as possible. Regardless, purchasing this Book can be seen as consent to the fact that both the publisher and the author of this book are in no way experts on the topics discussed within and that any recommendations or suggestions that are made herein are for entertainment purposes only. Professionals should be consulted as needed prior to undertaking any of the action endorsed herein.

This declaration is deemed fair and valid by both the American Bar Association and the Committee of Publishers Association and is legally binding throughout the United States.

Furthermore, the transmission, duplication, or reproduction of any of the following work including specific information will be considered an illegal act irrespective of if it is done electronically or in print. This extends to creating a secondary or tertiary copy of the work or a recorded copy and is only allowed with the express written consent from the Publisher. All additional right reserved.

The information in the following pages is broadly considered a truthful and accurate account of facts and as such, any inattention, use, or misuse of the information in question by the reader will render any resulting actions solely under their purview. There are no scenarios in which the publisher or the original author of this work can be in any fashion deemed liable for any hardship or damages that may befall them after undertaking information described herein.

Additionally, the information in the following pages is intended only for informational purposes and should thus be thought of as universal. As befitting its nature, it is presented without assurance regarding its prolonged validity or interim quality. Trademarks that are mentioned are done without written consent and can in no way be considered an endorsement from the trademark holder.

TABLE OF CONTENTS

TABLE OF CONTENTS 7
BREAKFAST 10
   Sweet and Sour Pan with Cashew Nuts 10
   Vegetarian Paleo Ratatouille 13
   Frittata with Spring Onions and Asparagus 15
   Apple Pastry 17
   Baked Maple Apple 19
   Apple-Raisin Cake 21
   Cinnamon-Apricot Bananas 23
   Meringue Crepes with Blueberry Custard Filling 25
   Chilled Cherry Soup 27
   Iced Orange Punch 29
   Meatless Borscht 31
   Sautéed Sweet 'N' Sour Beets 33
   Orange Beets 35
   Cabbage 'N' Potato Soup 37
   Eggplant Pesto 39
   Ratatouille 41
   Snowflakes 43
   Mild Cream Brussels Sprouts 44
   Brussels Sprouts Salad With Pears And Pomegranate 46
   Crowning Chicken Salad 48
LUNCH 51
   Cajun Steak and Veg Rice Jar Recipe 51
   Pesto Salmon Pasta Noodles Recipe 53
   Sri Lankan-Style Sweet Potato Curry Recipe 55
   Chicken Liver Along With Tomato Ragu Recipe 58
   Minted Lamb with a Couscous Salad Recipe 60
   Flax Seed Curd with Apple and Cucumber 62
   Green Omelet 64
DINNER 67
   Pan-Fried Salmon Burgers with Garlic and Greens 67
   Mushrooms Stuffed & Crab Paste 69
   Taco Pie 71

SNACKS & DESSERTS 74
- Apricot Oatmeal Cookies 74
- Raw Vegan Reese's Cups 76
- Raw Vegan Coffee Cashew Cream Cake 78
- Raw Vegan Chocolate Cashew Truffles 80
- Raw Vegan Double Almond Raw Chocolate Tart 81
- Raw Vegan Bounty Bars 83
- Raw Vegan Tartlets With Coconut Cream 86
- Raw Vegan "Peanut" Butter Truffles 88

SOUPS & STEWS 92
- Carrot Soup 92
- Chickpeas Stew 95
- Green Beans Stew 97
- Cauliflower and Walnut Soup 99
- Celery and Blue Cheese Soup 102
- Sweet Potato and Kale Soup 104
- Kale, Apple, and Fennel Soup 106
- Lentil Soup 108
- Spicy Pumpkin Soup 110
- French Onion Soup 112
- Creamy Broccoli and Kale Soup 114
- Creamy Asparagus Soup 117

BREAKFAST

Sweet and Sour Pan with Cashew Nuts

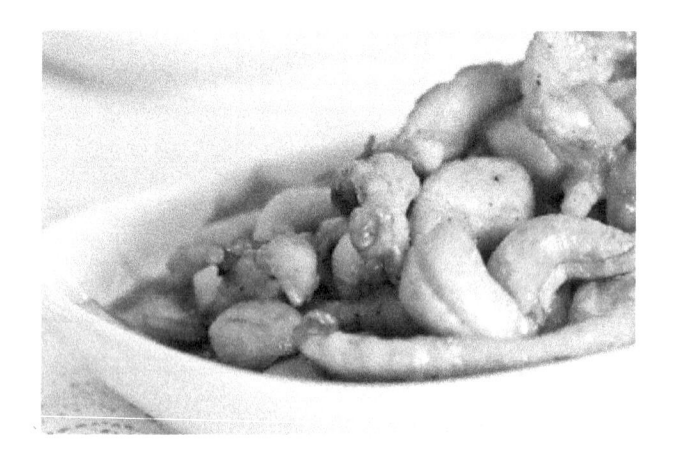

Preparation time: 30 minutes

Cooking time: 0 minutes

Servings: 2

Ingredients:

- 2 tablespoon Coconut oil
- 2 pieces Red onion
- 2 pieces yellow bell pepper
- 250 g White cabbage
- 150 g Pak choi
- 50 g Mung bean sprouts
- 4 pieces Pineapple slices
- 50 g Cashew nuts
- For the sweet and sour sauce:
- 60 ml Apple cider vinegar
- 4 tablespoon Coconut blossom sugar
- 11/2 tablespoon Tomato paste
- 1 teaspoon Coconut-Amines
- 2 teaspoon Arrowroot powder
- 75 ml Water

Directions:

1. Roughly cut the vegetables.

2. Mix the arrow root with five tablespoons of cold water into a paste.
3. Then put all the other ingredients for the sauce in a saucepan and add the arrowroot paste for binding.
4. Melt the coconut oil in a pan and fry the onion.
5. Add the bell pepper, cabbage, pak choi and bean sprouts and stir-fry until the vegetables become a little softer.
6. Add the pineapple and cashew nuts and stir a few more times.
7. Pour a little sauce over the wok dish and serve.

Nutrition: Calories: 573 Protein: 15.25 g Fat: 27.81 g Carbohydrates: 77.91 g

Vegetarian Paleo Ratatouille

Preparation time: 1 hour 10 minutes

Cooking time: 55 minutes

Servings: 2

Ingredients:

- 200 g Tomato cubes (can)
- 1 / 2 pieces Onion
- 2 cloves Garlic
- 1 / 4 teaspoon dried oregano
- 1 / 4 TL Chili flakes
- 2 tablespoon Olive oil
- 1 piece Eggplant
- 1 piece Zucchini
- 1 piece hot peppers
- 1 teaspoon dried thyme

Directions:

1. Preheat the oven to 180 ° C and lightly grease a round or oval shape.
2. Finely chop the onion and garlic.

3. Mix the tomato cubes with garlic, onion, oregano and chili flakes, season with salt and pepper and put on the bottom of the baking dish.
4. Use a mandolin, a cheese slicer or a sharp knife to cut the eggplant, zucchini and hot pepper into very thin slices.
5. Put the vegetables in a bowl (make circles, start at the edge and work inside).
6. Drizzle the remaining olive oil on the vegetables and sprinkle with thyme, salt and pepper.
7. Cover the baking dish with a piece of parchment paper and bake in the oven for 45 to 55 minutes.

Nutrition: Calories: 273 Protein: 5.66 g Fat: 14.49 g Carbohydrates: 35.81 g

Frittata with Spring Onions and Asparagus

Preparation time: 15 minutes

Cooking time: 10 minutes

Servings: 2

Ingredients:

- 5 pieces Egg
- 80 ml Almond milk
- 2 tablespoon Coconut oil
- 1 clove Garlic
- 100 g Asparagus tips
- 4 pieces Spring onions
- 1 teaspoon Tarragon
- 1 pinch Chili flakes

Directions:

1. Preheat the oven to 220 ° C.
2. Squeeze the garlic and finely chop the spring onions.
3. Whisk the eggs with the almond milk and season with salt and pepper.

4. Melt 1 tablespoon of coconut oil in a medium-sized cast iron pan and briefly fry the onion and garlic with the asparagus.
5. Remove the vegetables from the pan and melt the remaining coconut oil in the pan.
6. Pour in the egg mixture and half of the entire vegetable.
7. Place the pan in the oven for 15 minutes until the egg has solidified.
8. Then take the pan out of the oven and pour the rest of the egg with the vegetables into the pan.
9. Place the pan in the oven again for 15 minutes until the egg is nice and loose.
10. Sprinkle the tarragon and chili flakes on the dish before serving.

Nutrition: Calories: 464 kcal Protein: 24.23 g Fat: 37.84 g Carbohydrates: 7.33 g

Apple Pastry

Preparation time: 15 minutes

Cooking time: 30 minutes

Servings: 1

Ingredients:

- Three cups all-purpose flour
- Dash of salt
- Two teaspoons margarine
- One plain low-fat yogurt
- One small apple
- Dash each ground nutmeg and ground cinnamon
- Two teaspoons reduced-calorie apricot spread (16 calories per 2 teaspoons)

Directions:

1. In a small mixing bowl, combine flour and salt; with a pastry blender, or two knives used scissors-fashion, cut in margarine until the mixture resembles a coarse meal. Add yogurt and mix thoroughly. Form dough into a ball; wrap in plastic wrap and refrigerate for at least 1 hour (maybe kept in the refrigerator for up to 3 days).

2. Between 2 sheets of a wax paper roll dough, forming a 4/2-inch circle about 1/2. Inch thick. Carefully remove wax paper and place dough on foil or small cookie sheet—Preheat oven to 350°F.
3. Core, pare, and thinly slice apple; arrange slices decoratively over the dough and sprinkle with nutmeg and cinnamon. Bake until crust is golden, 20 to 30 minutes.
4. During the last few minutes, that pastry is baking, in a small metal measuring cup or other small flameproof container heat apricot spread; as soon as the pie is done, brush with a warm space.

Nutrition: 238 calories; 4 g protein; 8 g fat; 38 g carbohydrate; 228 mg sodium;1 mg cholesterol.

Baked Maple Apple

Preparation time: 10 minutes

Cooking time: 30 minutes

Servings: 2

Ingredients:

- Two small apples
- Two teaspoons reduced-calorie apricot
- Spread
- One teaspoon reduced-calorie maple-flavored syrup

Directions:

1. Remove the core from each apple to 1/2 inch from the bottom. Remove a thin strip of peel from around the center of each apple (this helps keep skin from bursting). Fill each apple with one teaspoon apricot spread and 1/2 teaspoon maple syrup. Place each apple upright in individual baking dish; cover dishes with foil and bake at 400°F until apples are tender, 25 to 30 minutes.

Nutrition: 75 calories; 0.2 g protein; 1 g fat; 19 g carbohydrate; 0.3 mg sodium;

Apple-Raisin Cake

Preparation time: 20 minutes

Cooking time: 50 minutes

Servings: 12

Ingredients:

- One teaspoon baking soda
- 1/2 cups applesauce (no sugar added)
- Two small Golden Delicious apples, cored, pared, and shredded
- 1 cup less 2 s raisins
- 2/4 cups self-rising flour
- 1 teaspoon ground cinnamon
- 1/2 teaspoon ground cloves 1/3 cup plus 2 teaspoons unsalted margarine
- 1/4 cup granulated sugar

Directions:

1. Spray an 8 x 8 x 2-inch baking pan with nonstick cooking spray and set aside. Into a medium bowl sift together flour, cinnamon, and cloves; set aside.

2. Preheat oven to 350°F. In a medium mixing bowl, using an electric mixer, cream margarine, add sugar and stir to combine. Stir baking soda into applesauce, and then add to margarine mixture and stir to combine; add sifted ingredients and, using an electric mixer on medium speed, beat until thoroughly combined. Fold in apples and raisins; pour batter into the sprayed pan and bake for 45 to 50 minutes (until cake is browned and a cake tester or toothpick, inserted in center, comes out dry). Remove cake from pan and cool on wire rack.

Nutrition: 151 calories; 2 g protein; 4 g fat; 28 g carbohydrate; 96 mg sodium;

Cinnamon-Apricot Bananas

Preparation time: 45 minutes

Cooking time: 40 minutes

Servings: 2

Ingredients:

- 4 graham crackers 2x2-inch 1 medium banana, peeled and cut in squares), made into crumbs half lengthwise
- 2 teaspoons shredded coconut
- 1/4 teaspoon ground cinnamon
- 1 plus 1 teaspoon reduced-calorie apricot spread (16 calories per 2 teaspoons)

Directions:

1. In small skillet combine crumbs, coconut, and cinnamon and toast lightly, being careful not to burn; transfer to a sheet of wax paper or a paper plate and set aside.
2. In the same skillet heat apricot spread until melted; remove from heat. Roll each banana half in a spread, then quickly roll in crumb mixture, pressing crumbs so that they adhere to the

banana; place coated halves on a plate, cover lightly, and refrigerate until chilled.
3. Variation: Coconut-Strawberry Bananas —Omit cinnamon and substitute reduced-calorie strawberry spread (16 calories per 2 teaspoons) for the apricot spread.

Nutrition: 130 calories; 2g protein; 2g fat; 29g carbohydrate; 95mg sodium;

Meringue Crepes with Blueberry Custard Filling

Preparation time: 10 minutes

Cooking time: 20 minutes

Servings: 4

Ingredients:

- 2 cups blueberries (reserve 8 berries for garnish)
- 1 cup evaporated skimmed milk
- 2 large eggs, separated
- 1 plus 1 teaspoon granulated sugar, divided
- 2 teaspoons each cornstarch
- Lemon juice

Directions:

1. In 1-quart saucepan, combine milk, egg yolks, and one sugar; cook over low heat, continually stirring, until slightly thickened and bubbles form around sides of the mixture. In a cup or small bowl dissolve cornstarch in lemon juice; gradually stir into milk mixture and cook, constantly stirring, until thick. Remove from heat and fold in blueberries; let cool.

2. Spoon Vs. of custard onto the center of each crepe and fold sides over filling to enclose; arrange crepes, seam-side down, in an 8 x 8 x 2-inch baking pan. In a small bowl, using an electric mixer on high speed beat egg whites until soft peaks form; add remaining teaspoon sugar, and continue beating until stiff peaks form.
3. Fill the pastry bag with egg whites and pipe an equal amount over each crepe (if pastry bag is not available, spoon egg whites over crepes); top each with a reserved blueberry and broil until meringue is lightly browned, 10 to 15 seconds. Serve immediately.

Nutrition: 300 calories; 16g protein; 6g fat; 45g carbohydrate; 180mg sodium;278mg cholesterol

Chilled Cherry Soup

Preparation time: 5 minutes

Cooking time: 5 minutes

Servings: 2

Ingredients:

- 20 large frozen pitted cherries (no sugar added)
- 1/2 cup water
- 1/2 teaspoons granulated sugar
- 2-inch cinnamon stick
- 1 strip lemon peel
- 2 s rose wine
- 1 teaspoon cornstarch
- 1/4 cup plain low-fat yogurt

Directions:

1. In a small saucepan, combine cherries, water, sugar, cinnamon stick, and lemon peel; bring to a boil. Reduce heat, cover, and let simmer for 20 minutes.
2. Remove and discard the cinnamon stick and lemon peel from a cherry mixture. In measuring cup or small bowl combine wine and cornstarch,

stirring to dissolve cornstarch; add to cherry mixture and, constantly stirring, bring to a boil. Reduce heat and let simmer until the mixture thickens.
3. In a heatproof bowl, stir yogurt until smooth; add cherry mixture and stir to combine. Cover with plastic wrap and refrigerate until well chilled

Nutrition: 98 calories; 2 g protein; 1 g fat; 19 g carbohydrate; 21 mg sodium; 2 mg cholesterol

Iced Orange Punch

Preparation time: 20 minutes

Cooking time: 0 minutes

Servings: 8

Ingredients:

- Ice Mold
- Club soda
- 1 lemon, sliced
- 1 lime, sliced
- Punch
- 1 quart each chilled orange juice (no sugar added), club soda, and diet ginger ale)

Directions:

1. To Prepare Ice Mold: Pour enough club soda into a 10- or 12-cup ring mold to fill mold; add lemon and lime slices, arranging them in an alternating pattern. Cover the mold and carefully transfer to freezer; freeze until solid.
2. To Prepare Punch: In a large punch bowl, combine juice and sodas. Remove ice mold from ring mold and float ice mold in a punch.

Nutrition: 56 calories; 1g protein; 0.1 g fat; 14 g carbohydrate; 35 mg sodium;

Meatless Borscht

Preparation time: 15 minutes

Cooking time: 45 minutes

Servings: 2

Ingredients:

- 1 teaspoon margarine
- 1 cup shredded green cabbage
- 1/4 cup chopped onion
- 1/4 cup sliced carrot
- 1 cup coarsely shredded pared
- 2 s tomato paste beets
- 1 lemon juice
- 2 cups of water
- 1/2 teaspoon granulated sugar
- 2 packets instant beef broth and 1 teaspoon pepper
- Seasoning mix
- 1/4 cup plain low-fat yogurt
- 1/2 bay leaf

Directions:

1. In 1 1/2-quart saucepan heat margarine until bubbly and hot; add onion and sauté until softened, 1 to 2 minutes. Add beets and toss to combine; add water, broth mix, and bay leaf and bring to a boil. Cover pan and cook over medium heat for 10 minutes; stir in remaining ingredients except for yogurt, cover, and let simmer until vegetables are tender about 25 minutes. Remove and discard bay leaf. Pour borscht into 2 soup bowls and top each portion with 2 s yogurt.

Nutrition: 120 calories; 5g protein; 3g fat; 21g carbohydrate;

982mg sodium;2mg cholesterol

Sautéed Sweet 'N' Sour Beets

Preparation time: 10 minutes

Cooking time: 10 minutes

Servings: 2

Ingredients:

- Serve hot or chilled.
- 2 teaspoons margarine
- 1 diced onion
- 1 cup drained canned small whole beets, cut into quarters
- 1 each lemon juice and water
- 1 teaspoon each salt and pepper
- Dash granulated sugar substitute

Directions:

1. In small nonstick skillet heat margarine over medium-high heat until bubbly and hot; add onion and sauté until softened, 1 to 2 minutes. Reduce heat to low and add remaining ingredients; cover pan and cook, stirring once, for 5 minutes longer.

Nutrition: 70 calories; 1g protein; 4g fat; 9g carbohydrate; 385 mg sodium;

Orange Beets

Preparation time: 10 minutes

Cooking time: 10 minutes

Servings: 2

Ingredients:

- 1 /2 teaspoons lemon juice
- 1 teaspoon cornstarch Dash salt
- 1 teaspoon orange marmalade
- 1 cup peeled and sliced cooked beets
- 2 teaspoons margarine
- 1 teaspoon firmly packed brown
- Sugar 1/4 cup orange juice (no sugar added)

Directions:

1. In a 1-quart saucepan (not aluminum or cast-iron), combine beets, margarine, and sugar; cook over low heat, continually stirring until margarine and sugar are melted.
2. In 1-cup measure or small bowl combine juices, cornstarch, and salt, stirring to dissolve cornstarch; pour over beet mixture and,

constantly stirring, bring to a boil. Continue cooking and stirring
3. Until the mixture thickens.
4. Reduce heat, add marmalade, and stir until combined. Remove from heat and let cool slightly; cover and refrigerate for at least 1 hour. Reheat before serving.

Nutrition: 99 calories; 1g protein; 4g fat; 16g carbohydrate; 146mg sodium;

Cabbage 'N' Potato Soup

Preparation time: 10 minutes

Cooking time: 40 minutes

Servings: 4

Ingredients:

- This soup freezes well; for easy portion control, freeze in pre-measured servings.
- 2 teaspoons vegetable oil
- 4 cups shredded green cabbage
- 1 cup sliced onions
- 1 garlic clove, minced
- 3 cups of water
- 6 ounces peeled potato, sliced
- 1 cup each sliced carrot and tomato puree
- 4 packets instant beef broth and seasoning mix
- 1 each bay leaf and whole clove

Directions:

1. In 2-quart saucepan heat oil, add cabbage, onions, and garlic and sauté over medium heat, frequently stirring, until cabbage is soft, about 10 minutes. Reduce heat to low and add remaining

ingredients; cook until vegetables are tender, about 30 minutes. Remove and discard bay leaf and clove before serving.

Nutrition: 119 calories; 4 g protein; 3 g fat; 22 g carbohydrate; 900 mg sodium,

Eggplant Pesto

Preparation time: 15 minutes

Cooking time: 30 minutes

Servings: 2

Ingredients:

- 1 medium eggplant (about 1 pound), cut crosswise into thick rounds
- Dash salt
- Fresh basil and grated Parmesan cheese
- 1 olive oil
- 1 small garlic clove, mashed
- Dash freshly ground pepper

Directions:

1. On 10 X 15-inch nonstick baking sheet arrange eggplant slices in a single layer; sprinkle with salt and bake at 425°F. Until easily pierced with a fork, about 30 minutes.
2. In a small bowl, combine remaining ingredients; spread an equal amount of mixture over each eggplant slice. Transfer slices to I1/2-quart

casserole, return to oven, and bake until heated, about 10 minutes longer.

Nutrition: 144 calories; 5g protein; 9g fat; 14g carbohydrate; 163mg sodium;4mg cholesterol

Ratatouille

Preparation time: 15 minutes

Cooking time: 30 minutes

Servings: 4

Ingredients:

- 1 plus 1 teaspoon olive oil
- 1 cup each sliced onions and red or green bell peppers
- 3 garlic cloves, chopped
- 4 cups cubed eggplant (1-inch cubes)
- 1/2 cups canned Italian tomatoes,
- Chopped 1 cup sliced zucchini
- 3 s chopped fresh basil or 2 teaspoons dried
- 1 teaspoon salt
- Dash freshly ground pepper

Directions:

1. In 12-inch skillet heat oil over medium heat; add onions, bell peppers, and garlic and sauté until vegetables are tender-crisp. Add remaining ingredients and stir to combine. Reduce heat,

cover, and let simmer until vegetables are tender, 20 to 25 minutes.

Nutrition: 123 calories; 4g protein; 5g fat; 18g carbohydrate; 666mg sodium

Snowflakes

Preparation time: 15 minutes

Cooking time: 10 minutes

Servings: 1

Ingredients:

- Won ton wrappers
- Oil to frying
- Powdered sugar

Directions:

1. Cut won ton wrappers just like you'd a snowflake
2. Heat oil. When hot, add wonton, fry for approximately 30 seconds then flip over.
3. Drain on a paper towel and dust with powdered sugar.

Nutrition: Calories: 96 Net carbs: 24.1g Fat: 0.6g Fiber: 5.3g Protein: 2.8g

Mild Cream Brussels Sprouts

Preparation time: 10 minutes

Cooking time: 20 minutes

Servings: 3

Ingredients:

- 1 kg of Brussels sprouts
- 150 ml vegetable broth
- 50 g butter
- 1 onion
- 150 g cream
- 1-2 light sauce binders
- Salt, pepper, nutmeg, sugar

Directions:

1. Clean the Brussels sprouts by removing the outer leaves and washing them well. Halve large florets and cut the stalk crosswise. Cook with a little sugar in boiling salted water for a good ten to twelve minutes. Drain and drain.
2. Finely dice the onion and fry in the butter. Then add the Brussels sprouts and let them steam briefly. Then deglaze with the cream and the

vegetable broth and simmer for two minutes on a low flame.
3. Now stir in the gravy until the creamy vegetables have a creamy consistency. Season with salt, pepper and nutmeg and enjoy.

Nutrition: Calories: 162 Net carbs: 42.4g Fat: 0.2g Fiber: 3.9g Protein: 0.4g

Brussels Sprouts Salad With Pears And Pomegranate

Preparation time: 30 minutes

Cooking time: 30 minutes

Servings: 4

Ingredients:

- 400 g Brussels sprouts
- 4 white wine vinegar
- 4 walnut oil
- 1 shallot
- 80 g walnuts
- 1 pomegranate
- 1 lemon
- 2 pears
- Salt

Directions:

1. Clean the Brussels sprouts and remove the outer leaves. Remove the stalk and pluck off the individual leaves of the florets. Then wash them, add a little salt and pour hot water over them for five minutes. Then drain well.

2. Mix white wine vinegar, walnut oil, salt, and pepper into a vinaigrette. Add the previously diced shallot and the Brussels sprouts leave. Let everything steep for a quarter of an hour.
3. Roughly chop the walnuts and roast them in a pan without fat.
4. Remove the pomegranate seeds from the fruit and squeeze the juice from the lemon.
5. The bulb you wash and hobbles then follow with a vegetable slicer into thin slices. Drizzle with lemon juice.
6. Now put everything together in a bowl, season to taste and welcome the autumn in a delicious way.

Nutrition: Calories: 207 Net carbs: 4.7g Fat: 10.2g Protein: 22.4g

Crowning Chicken Salad

Preparation time: 30 minutes

Cooking time: 45 minutes

Servings: 5

Ingredients:

- 600 grams of boneless roasted chicken and chopped
- 25 grams of shallots, finely chopped
- 10 grams of butter
- 1/2 curry powder
- 1/2 finely chopped red chili
- 5 grams of tomato paste
- 80 ml white wine
- 1 bay leaf
- 50 ml of chicken broth
- 15 grams of apricot jam
- 70 grams of mayonnaise
- 20 ml of milk cream
- 20 grams of Fraiche cream
- 10 ml of lemon juice
- 5 grams of chopped cilantro
- 1 pinch of salt

- 1 pinch of black pepper
- To present;
- 20 grams of rolled almonds, toasted
- 4 chopped scallions
- Mixed lettuces

Directions:

1. In a medium casserole, melt the butter and poach the shallots with salt and pepper for about 3 minutes. Add the bay leaf, curry powder and tomato paste. We cook for another 3 minutes.
2. Next, add the wine and reduce until it is almost dry, then add the apricot jam and chicken broth. Reduce to medium heat until it reaches a thick consistency of syrup and let cool.
3. Once the mixture has cooled, we mix all the remaining ingredients, add the chicken once the liquid has emulsified. Let marinate for 2 hours.
4. To serve, we place a lettuce base on each plate. Add the coronation chicken on top and sprinkle with spring almonds and spring onions to finish.

Nutrition: Calories: 381 Net carbs: 4.1g Fat: 27.7g Fiber: 0.6g Protein: 27.6g

LUNCH

Cajun Steak and Veg Rice Jar Recipe

Preparation time: 20 minutes

Cooking time: 30 minutes

Servings: 2

Ingredients:

- 1 tablespoon vegetable oil
- 1 celery stick, finely chopped
- 3 large carrots, sliced into rounds
- 250g frozen chopped mixed peppers
- 4 spring onions, chopped, green and white parts split
- 500g 5 percent beef mince
- 2 teaspoon seasoning
- 1 teaspoon tomato purée
- 2 x 250g packs ready-cooked long-grain rice

Directions:

1. Heat the oil in a large, shallow skillet over moderate heat. Add the carrots, celery, peppers, and snowy areas of the nuts. Cook for 10 minutes before the veg is beginning to soften.
2. Insert the mince, season liberally, and cook for 10 minutes before mince is browned and start to really go crispy.
3. Insert the Cajun seasoning and tomato purée; stir fry to coat the mince. Hint inside the rice combined with 4 tablespoons of plain water. Stir to completely unite heat and heat until the rice is hot. Scatter on the rest of the spring onion before serving.

Nutrition: Carbohydrate 53.1gram Protein 32.8gram Fiber 8.3gram

Pesto Salmon Pasta Noodles Recipe

Preparation time: 20 minutes

Cooking time: 30 minutes

Servings: 2

Ingredients:

- 350g penne
- 2 x 212g tins cherry salmon, drained
- 1 lemon, zested and juiced
- 190g jar green pesto
- 250g package cherry tomatoes halved
- 100g bunch spring onions, finely chopped
- 125g package reduced-fat mozzarella

Directions:

1. Pre heats the oven to Windows 7, 220°C, buff 200°C. Boil the pasta for 5 minutes. Drain, reserving 100ml drinking water.
2. Meanwhile, at a 2ltr ovenproof dish, then mix the salmon, lemon zest, and juice, then pesto (booking 2 tablespoons)berries and half of the spring onions; season.

3. Mix the pasta and reserved cooking water to the dish. Mix the allowed pesto using 1 tablespoon water and then drizzle on the pasta. Gently within the mozzarella, top with the rest of the spring onions and bake for 25 minutes until golden.

Nutrition: Carbohydrate 72.2gram Protein 43.2gram Fiber 2.6gram

Sri Lankan-Style Sweet Potato Curry Recipe

Preparation time: 10 minutes

Cooking time: 25 minutes

Servings: 3

Ingredients:

- 1/2 onion, roughly sliced
- 3 garlic cloves, roughly sliced
- 25g sliced ginger, chopped and peeled
- 15g fresh coriander stalks and leaves split leaves sliced
- Two 1/2 tablespoon moderate tikka curry powder
- 60g package cashew nuts
- 1 tablespoon olive oil
- 500g Redmere Farms sweet potatoes, peeled and cut into 3cm balls
- 400ml tin Isle Sun Coconut-milk
- 1/2 vegetable stock block, created as much as 300ml
- 200g Grower's Harvest long-grain rice
- 300g frozen green beans

- 150g Redmere Farms lettuce

Directions:

1. Set the onion, ginger, garlic, coriander stalks tikka powder along with half of the cashew nuts in a food processor. Insert 2 tablespoons water and blitz to a chunky paste.
2. At a large skillet, warm the oil over moderate heat. Insert the paste and cook, stirring for 5 minutes. Bring the sweet potatoes, stir, and then pour into the coconut milk and stock. Bring to the simmer and boil for 25-35 minutes before the sweet potatoes are tender.
3. Meanwhile, cook the rice pack directions. Toast the rest of the cashews at a dry skillet.
4. Stir the beans into the curry and then simmer for two minutes. Insert the lettuce in handfuls, allowing each to simmer before adding the following; simmer for 1 minute. Bring the lemon juice, to taste, & the majority of the coriander leaves. Scatter on the remaining coriander and cashews, then use the rice and lemon wedges.

Nutrition: Carbohydrate 84.2gram Protein 12.1gram Fiber 8.4gram

Chicken Liver Along With Tomato Ragu Recipe

Preparation time: 20 minutes

Cooking time: 60 minutes

Servings: 2

Ingredients:

- 2 tablespoon olive oil
- 1 onion, finely chopped
- 2 carrots scrubbed and simmer
- 4 garlic cloves, finely chopped
- 1/4 x 30g pack fresh ginger, stalks finely chopped, leaves ripped
- 380g package poultry livers, finely chopped, and almost any sinew removed and lost
- 400g tin Grower's Harvest chopped berries
- 1 chicken stock cube, created around 300ml
- 1/2 tsp. caster sugar
- 300g penne
- 1/4 Suntrail Farms lemon, juiced

Directions:

1. Heat 1 tablespoon oil in a large skillet, over a low-medium heating system. Fry the onion and carrots to 10 minutes, stirring periodically. Stir in the ginger and garlic pops and cook 2 minutes more. Transfer into a bowl set aside.
2. Twist the pan into high heat and then add the oil. Bring the chicken livers and simmer for 5 minutes until browned. Pour the onion mix to the pan and then stir in the tomatoes, sugar, and stock. Season, bring to the boil, and then simmer for 20 minutes until reduced and thickened and also the liver is cooked through. Meanwhile, cook pasta to package Direction.
3. Taste the ragu and put in a second pinch of sugar more seasoning, if needed. Put in a squeeze of lemon juice to taste and stir in two of the ripped basil leaves. Divide the pasta between four bowls, then spoon across the ragu and top with the rest of the basil.

Nutrition: Carbohydrate 69.1gram Protein 25.8gram Fiber 3.3gram

Minted Lamb with a Couscous Salad Recipe

Preparation time: 10 minutes

Cooking time: 20 minutes

Servings: 1

Ingredients:

- 75g Cous-cous
- 1/2 chicken stock block, composed to 125ml
- 30g pack refreshing flat-leaf parsley, sliced
- 3 mint sprigs, leaves picked and sliced
- 1 tablespoon olive oil
- 200g pack suspended BBQ minted lamb leg beans, De-frosted
- 200g lettuce berries, sliced
- 1/4 tsp., sliced
- 1 spring onion, sliced
- Pinch of ground cumin
- 1/2 lemon, zested and juiced
- 50g reduced-fat salad cheese
- Each Serving comprises

Directions:

1. Place the couscous into a heatproof bowl and then pour on the inventory. Cover and set aside for 10 minutes, then fluff with a fork and stir in the herbs.
2. Meanwhile, rub a little oil within the lamb steaks and season. Cook to package Direction then slit.
3. Mix the tomatoes, cucumber and spring onion into the couscous with the oil, the cumin, and lemon juice and zest. Crumble on the salad and serve with the bunny.

Nutrition: Carbohydrate 41.1gram Protein 33.8gram Fiber 4.1gram

Flax Seed Curd with Apple and Cucumber

Preparation time: 10 minutes

Cooking time: 10 minutes

Ingredients:

- 150 Grams of herb curd ("Almased vital food")
- 150 Grams of cream cheese ("Buko with Skyr")
- 1 Tablespoons linseed oil
- 3rd Tablespoons of lemon juice
- 2nd Tablespoons flaxseed (crushed, see merchandise knowledge)
- 30th Grams
- Seasoned Salt
- Pepper (freshly ground)
- 3rd Tablespoons chives (rolls, fresh or frozen)
- 1 Apple (150 g)
- 1 Mini cucumber (80 g)
- Linseed (for sprinkling)
- Chives (for sprinkling)

Directions:

1. Mix the herb curd, "Buko with Skyr", linseed oil, lemon juice, linseed and "Almased" and season with herb salt and pepper. Stir in chives.
2. Rinse the apple and cucumber hot and grate dry. Quarter the apple, core it and cut it into thick slices, cucumber into long sticks.
3. Arrange the quark, apple and cucumber and sprinkle with flax seeds and chives.

Nutrition: Per Servings: 345 kcal, 17g fat, 22g carbohydrates, 26g protein

Green Omelet

Preparation time: 10 min

Cooking time: 5 min

Servings: 1

Ingredients:

- 2 large eggs, at room temperature
- 1 shallot, peeled and chopped
- Handful arugula
- 3 sprigs of parsley, chopped
- 1 tsp. extra virgin olive oil
- Salt and black pepper

Directions:

1. Beat the eggs in a small bowl and set aside. Sauté the shallot for 5 minutes with a bit of the oil, on low-medium heat. Pour the eggs in the pans, stirring the mixture for just a second.
2. The eggs on a medium heat, and tip the pan just enough to let the loose egg run underneath after about one minute on the burner. Add the greens, herbs, and the seasonings to the top side as it is still soft. TIP: You do not even have to flip it, as

you can just cook the egg slowly egg as is well (being careful as to not burn).

Nutrition: Calories: 448.1.Total Fat 37 g 56 % Saturated Fat 12.8 g 63 % Cholesterol 665 mg 221 % Sodium 316.7 mg 13 %

Total Carbohydrate 8 g 2 % Dietary Fiber 1.7 g 6 % Sugars 2.4 g 9 % Protein 22.9 g 45 %

DINNER

Pan-Fried Salmon Burgers with Garlic and Greens

Preparation Time: 30 minutes

Cooking Time: 30 minutes+ 1 hours to chill

Servings: 4

Ingredients:

- 1 lb. boneless Pacific salmon filet, skin removed
- 2 eggs, lightly beaten
- Pinch salt and pepper
- 2 tbsp. onion minced
- ½ cup homemade or Keto-friendly mayonnaise
- 1 clove garlic, minced
- A handful of fresh cilantros, minced
- 2 tbsp. coconut oil
- 12 oz. greens, such as spinach, arugula, or mixed

Directions:

1. Finely chop the salmon with a sharp chef's knife into ⅛"- ¼" pieces.
2. Mix with the egg, salt, pepper, and onion and form into four patties.
3. Chill for 1 hour.
4. Meanwhile, whisk together the mayonnaise with the garlic and cilantro.
5. Chill.
6. Heat the coconut oil in a large skillet and add the burgers.
7. Cook for 2-3 minutes per side, until opaque throughout.
8. Serve on a bed of greens topped with the garlic

Nutrition: Calories 195

Mushrooms Stuffed & Crab Paste

Preparation Time: 15 minutes

Cooking Time: 20 minutes

Servings: 15

Ingredients

- 20 ounces/566 grams mushrooms (about 20 mushrooms)
- 2 tablespoons parmesan cheese
- 1 tablespoon parsley (fresh, chopped)
- Salt
- For filling
- 4 ounces/100 grams cream cheese
- 4 ounces crab meat (chopped)
- 5 garlic cloves (minced)
- 1 teaspoon oregano
- ½ teaspoon paprika
- ½ teaspoon pepper
- ¼ teaspoon salt

Directions:

1. Preheat the oven to 400°F/200°C. Put parchment paper over the baking sheet.

2. Remove the stems from the mushrooms. Put the mushroom heads over the baking sheet (not too close to each other). Sprinkle with salt.
3. In a bowl, mix the filling ingredients. (There should be no lumps of cream cheese.) With a teaspoon, carefully stuff the mushroom caps with this cheese mix.
4. Sprinkle parmesan on top of each mushroom head.
5. Bake for half an hour or until the mushrooms are soft and the parmesan cheese is brownish in color.

Nutrition: Calories 34.1g Cholesterol 4.7mg Carbohydrate 2.7g Protein 5.0g

Taco Pie

Preparation Time: 20 minutes

Cooking Time: 10 minutes

Servings: 8

Ingredients

- 1-pound ground beef
- 3 tablespoons taco seasoning
- 6 eggs
- 1 cup heavy cream
- 2 garlic cloves (chopped)
- ½ teaspoon salt
- ¼ teaspoon pepper
- 1 cup cheddar cheese (shredded or grated)

Directions:

1. Preheat the oven to 350°F/180°C.
2. Grease a ceramic baking pan.
3. In another pot, cook the beef until it gets brown (medium heat, for seven minutes).
4. Put taco seasoning over the meat and stir well. Lower the heat and let it cook for a couple of minutes. (The sauce should thicken.)

5. Put the beef in the ceramic pan.
6. In another bowl, mix the eggs, cream, salt, pepper, and garlic. Pour this mix over the beef.
7. Top with cheese and bake for half an hour.
8. Once baked, take it out of the oven. Let it sit for a few minutes, then serve.
9. Decorate with sour cream, avocado, or other toppings of your choice.

Nutrition: Calories: 226.6 Total Fat: 9.8 g Protein: 19.0 g Saturated Fat: 3.0 g

SNACKS & DESSERTS

Apricot Oatmeal Cookies

Preparation time: 10 minutes

Cooking time: 40 minutes

Servings: 7

Ingredients:

- 1/2 cup (1 stick) butter, softened
- 2/3 cup light brown sugar packed
- 1 egg
- 3/4 cup all-purpose flour
- 1/2 teaspoon baking soda
- 1/2 teaspoon vanilla extract
- 1/2 teaspoon cinnamon
- 1/4 teaspoon salt
- 1 teaspoon 1/2 cups chopped oats
- 3/4 cup yolks
- 1/4 cup sliced apricots
- 1/3 cup slivered almonds

Directions:

1. Preheat oven to 350°.
2. In a big bowl combine with the butter, sugar, and egg until smooth.
3. In another bowl whisk the flour, baking soda, cinnamon, and salt together.
4. Stir the dry ingredients to the butter-sugar bowl.
5. Now stir in the oats, raisins, apricots, and almonds.
6. I heard on the web that in this time, it's much better to cool with the dough (therefore, your biscuits are thicker)

Nutrition: Calories: 196 Net carbs: 30g Fat: 8.1g Fiber: 0.5g Protein: 3g

Raw Vegan Reese's Cups

Preparation time: 10 minutes

Cooking time: 35 minutes

Servings: 4

Ingredients:

- "Peanut" butter filling
- ½ cup sunflower seeds butter
- ½ cup almond butter
- 1 raw honey
- 2 melted coconut oil
- Super foods chocolate part:
- ½ cup cacao powder
- 2 raw honey
- 1/3 cup of coconut oil (melted)

Directions:

1. Mix the "peanut" butter filling ingredients.
2. Put a spoonful of the mixture into each muffin cup.
3. Refrigerate.
4. Mix super foods chocolate ingredients.

5. Put a spoonful of the super foods chocolate mixture over the "peanut" butter mixture. Freeze!

Nutrition: Calories: 549 Net carbs: 54g Fat: 31.7g Fiber: 2.1g Protein: 11.8g

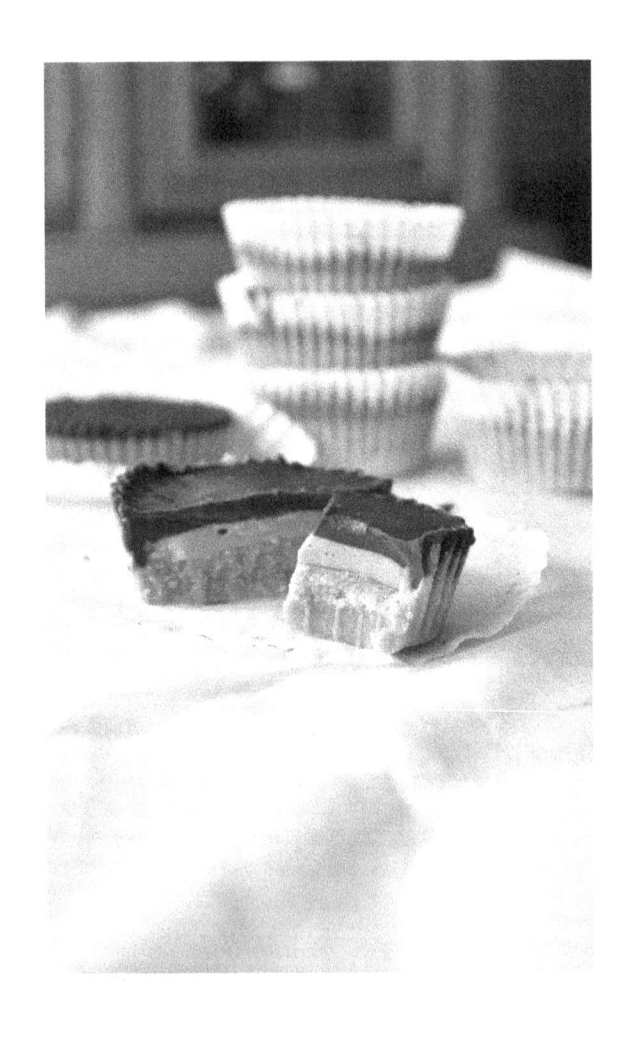

Raw Vegan Coffee Cashew Cream Cake

Preparation time: 10 minutes

Cooking time: 35 minutes

Servings: 4

Ingredients:

- Coffee cashew cream
- 2 cups raw cashews
- 1 teaspoon of ground vanilla bean
- 3 melted coconut oil
- ¼ cup raw honey
- 1/3 cup very strong coffee or triple espresso shot

Directions:

1. Blend all ingredients for the cream, pour it onto the crust and refrigerate.
2. Garnish with coffee beans.

Nutrition: Calories: 94 Net carbs: 4.4g Fat: 7.9g Fiber: 0.3g Protein: 2.8g

Raw Vegan Chocolate Cashew Truffles

Preparation time: 10 minutes

Cooking time: 35 minutes

Servings: 4

Ingredients:

- 1 cup ground cashews
- 1 teaspoon of ground vanilla bean
- ½ cup of coconut oil
- ¼ cup raw honey
- 2 flax meal
- 2 hemp hearts
- 2 cacao powder

Directions:

1. Mix all ingredients and make truffles. Sprinkle coconut flakes on top.

Nutrition: Calories: 87 Net carbs: 6g Fat: 6.5g Fiber: 0.5g Protein: 2.3g

Raw Vegan Double Almond Raw Chocolate Tart

Preparation time: 10 minutes

Cooking time: 35 minutes

Servings: 4

Ingredients:

- 1½ cups of raw almonds
- ¼ cup of coconut oil, melted
- 1 raw honey or royal jelly
- 8 ounces dark chocolate, chopped
- 1 cup of coconut milk
- ½ cup unsweetened shredded coconut

Directions:

1. Crust:
2. Ground almonds and add melted coconut oil, raw honey and combine.
3. Using a spatula, spread this mixture into the tart or pie pan.
4. Filling:
5. Put the chopped chocolate in a bowl, heat coconut milk and pour over chocolate and whisk together.

6. Pour filling into tart shell.
7. Refrigerate.
8. Toast almond slivers chips and sprinkle over tart.

Nutrition: Calories: 101 Net carbs: 3.4g Fat: 9.4g Fiber: 0.6g Protein: 2.4g

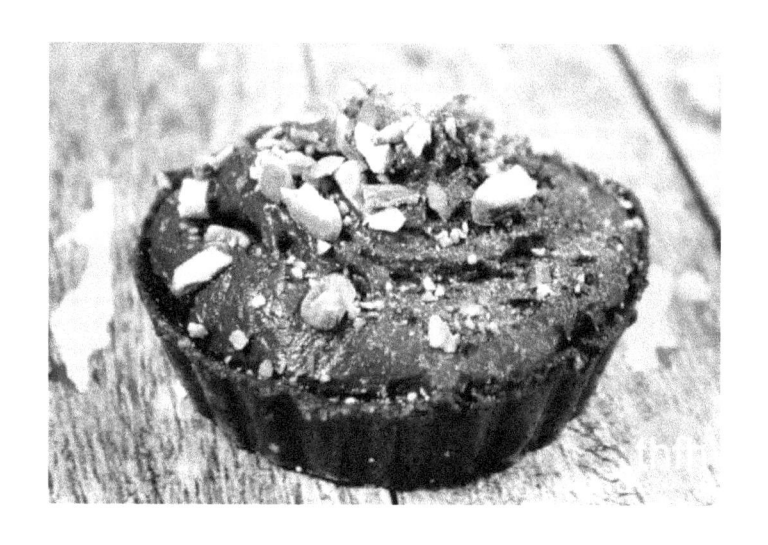

Raw Vegan Bounty Bars

Preparation time: 10 minutes

Cooking time: 35 minutes

Servings: 4

Ingredients:

- "Peanut" butter filling
- 2 cups desiccated coconut
- 3 coconut oil - melted
- 1 cup of coconut cream - full fat
- 4 of raw honey
- 1 teaspoon ground vanilla bean
- Pinch of sea salt
- Super foods chocolate part:
- ½ cup cacao powder
- 2 raw honey
- 1/3 cup of coconut oil (melted)

Directions:

1. Mix coconut oil, coconut cream, and honey, vanilla and salt.
2. Pour over desiccated coconut and mix well.

3. Mold coconut mixture into balls, small bars similar to bounty and freeze.
4. Or pour the whole mixture into a tray, freeze and cut into small bars.
5. Make super foods chocolate mixture, warm it up and dip frozen coconut into the chocolate and put on a tray and freeze again.

Nutrition: Calories: 70 Net carbs: 6.7g Fat: 4.3g Fiber: 0.2g Protein: 1g

Raw Vegan Tartlets With Coconut Cream

Preparation time: 10 minutes

Cooking time: 35 minutes

Servings: 4

Ingredients:

- Pudding:
- 1 avocado
- 2 coconut oil
- 2 raw honey
- 2 cacao powder
- 1 teaspoon ground vanilla bean
- Pinch of salt
- ¼ cup almond milk, as needed

Directions:

1. Blend all the ingredients in the food processor until smooth and thick.
2. Spread evenly into tartlet crusts.
3. Optionally, put some goji berries on top of the pudding layer.

4. Make the coconut cream, spread it on top of the pudding layer, and put back in the fridge overnight.
5. Serve with one blueberry on top of each tartlet.

Nutrition: Calories: 200 Net carbs: 25.2g Fat: 4.3g Fiber: 4.6g Protein: 12.8g

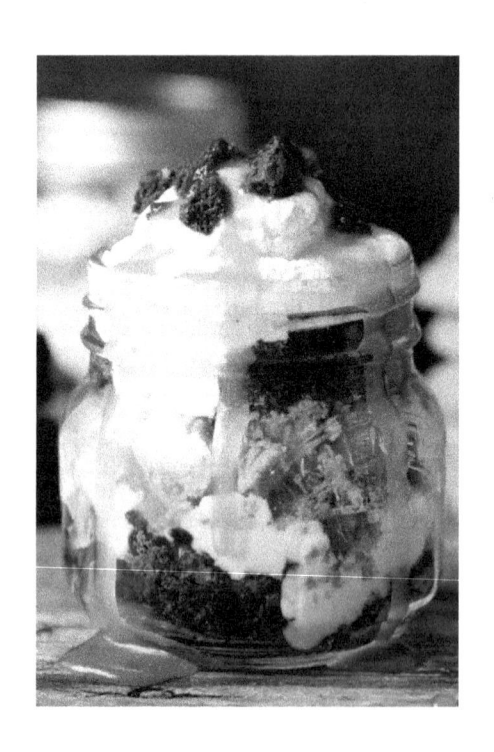

Raw Vegan "Peanut" Butter Truffles

Preparation time: 10 minutes

Cooking time: 30 minutes

Servings: 4

Ingredients:

- 5 sunflower seed butter
- 1 coconut oil
- 1 raw honey
- 1 teaspoon ground vanilla bean
- ¾ cup almond flour
- 1 flaxseed meal
- Pinch of salt
- 1 cacao butter
- Hemp hearts (optional)
- ¼ cup super-foods chocolate

Directions:

1. Mix until all ingredients are incorporated.
2. Roll the dough into 1-inch balls, place them on parchment paper and refrigerate for half an hour (yield about 14 truffles).

3. Dip each truffle in the melted super foods chocolate, one at the time.
4. Place them back on the pan with parchment paper or coat them in cocoa powder or coconut flakes.

Nutrition: Calories: 94 Net carbs: 3.1g Fat: 8g Fiber: 1g Protein: 4g

SOUPS & STEWS

Carrot Soup

Preparation Time: 10 minutes

Cooking Time: 35 minutes

Servings: 6

Ingredients:

- 5 cups vegetable broth
- 4 carrots, peeled
- 1 teaspoon dried thyme
- ½ teaspoon ground cumin
- 1 teaspoon salt
- 1 ½ cup potatoes, chopped
- 1 tablespoon olive oil
- ½ teaspoon ground black pepper
- 1 tablespoon lemon juice

- 1/3 cup fresh parsley, chopped
- 1 chili pepper, chopped
- 1 tablespoon tomato paste
- 1 tablespoon sour cream

Directions:

1. Line the baking tray with baking paper. Put sweet potatoes and carrot on the tray and sprinkle with olive oil and salt. Bake the vegetables for 25 minutes at 365F.

2. Meanwhile, pour the vegetable broth into the pan and bring it to boil. Add dried thyme, ground cumin, chopped chili pepper, and tomato paste.

3. When the vegetables are cooked, add them to the pan. Boil the vegetables until they are soft. Then blend the mixture with the help of the blender until smooth.

4. Simmer it for 2 minutes and add lemon juice. Stir well. Then add sour cream and chopped parsley. Stir well. Simmer the soup for 3 minutes more. Serve.

Nutrition: Calories: 123 Fat: 4.1 g Carbohydrates: 16.4 g Protein: 5.3 g

Chickpeas Stew

Preparation Time: 10 minutes

Cooking Time: 40 minutes

Servings: 4

Ingredients:

- 1 teaspoon olive oil
- 1 cup chickpeas, soaked within 8 hours and drained
- 4 garlic cloves, minced
- 1 yellow onion, chopped
- 1 green chili pepper, chopped
- 1 teaspoon coriander, ground
- ½ teaspoon cumin, ground
- ½ teaspoon sweet paprika
- 2 tomatoes, chopped
- 1 and ½ cups low-sodium veggie stock
- A pinch of black pepper

- 3 cups spinach leaves

- 1 tablespoon lemon juice

Directions:

1. Heat a pot with the oil over medium heat, add garlic, onion, and chili pepper, stir, and cook for 5 minutes. Add coriander, cumin, paprika, and black pepper, stir, and cook for 5 minutes more.

2. Add chickpeas, tomatoes, stock, and lemon juice stir, cover the pot, cook over medium heat for 25 minutes, add spinach, cook for 5 minutes more, divide into bowls, and serve.

Nutrition: Calories: 270 Fat: 7 g Carbohydrates: 14 g Protein: 9 g

Green Beans Stew

Preparation Time: 10 minutes

Cooking Time: 25 minutes

Servings: 4

Ingredients:

- 2 tablespoons olive oil
- 2 carrots, chopped
- 1 yellow onion, chopped
- 20 ounces green beans
- 2 garlic cloves, minced
- 7 ounces canned tomatoes, chopped
- 5 cups low-sodium veggie stock
- A pinch of black pepper
- 1 tablespoon parsley, chopped

Directions:

1. Heat a pot with the oil, over medium heat, add onion, stir, and cook for 5 minutes. Add carrots,

green beans, garlic, tomatoes, black pepper, and stock, stir, cover, and simmer over medium heat for 20 minutes. Add parsley, divide into bowls, and serve for lunch.

Nutrition: Calories: 281 Fat: 5 g Carbohydrates: 14 g Protein: 11 g

Cauliflower and Walnut Soup

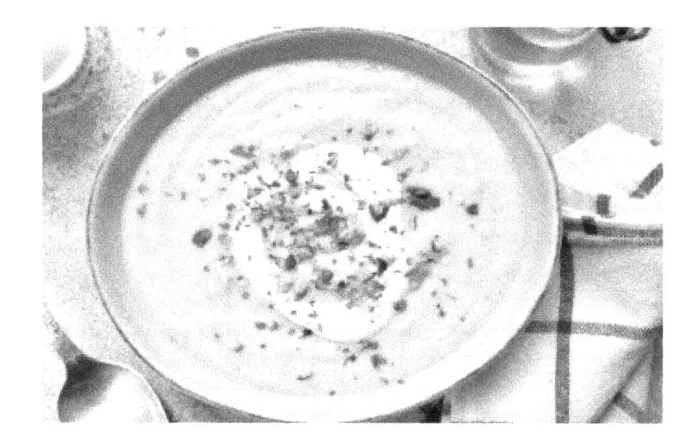

Preparation Time: 10 minutes

Cooking Time: 15 minutes

Servings: 4.

Ingredients:

- 450g (1lb) cauliflower, chopped
- 8 walnut halves, chopped
- 1 red onion, chopped
- 900mls (1½ pints) vegetable stock (broth)
- 100mls (3½ Fl oz) double cream (heavy cream)
- ½ teaspoon turmeric
- 1 tablespoon olive oil

Directions:

1. Warm oil in a saucepan, add the cauliflower and red onion, and cook for 4 minutes, stirring continuously. Pour in the stock (broth), bring to the boil, and cook for 15 minutes.

2. Stir in the walnuts, double cream, and turmeric. Process the soup until smooth and creamy Using

a food processor or hand blender. Serve into bowls and top off with a dash of chopped walnuts.

Nutrition: Calories: 244 Fat: 23g Carbs: 9g Protein: 5g

Celery and Blue Cheese Soup

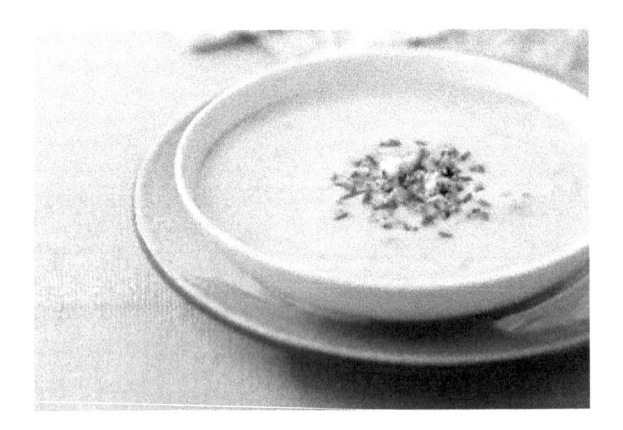

Preparation Time: 15 minutes

Cooking Time: 15 minutes

Servings: 4

Ingredients:

- 125g (4oz) blue cheese
- 25g (1oz) butter
- 1 head of celery (approx. 650g)
- 1 red onion, chopped
- 900mls (1½ pints) chicken stock (broth)
- 150mls (5fl oz) single cream

Directions:

1. Warm butter in a saucepan, add the onion and celery, and cook until the vegetables have softened. Pour in the stock, bring to the boil, then reduce the heat and simmer for 15 minutes. Pour in the cream and stir in the cheese until it has melted. Serve and eat straight away.

Nutrition: Calories: 341 Fat: 13.6g Carbs: 32g Protein: 18g

Sweet Potato and Kale Soup

Preparation Time: 10 minutes

Cooking Time: 30 minutes

Servings: 4

Ingredients:

- 1 medium red onion
- 1 garlic clove
- 2 medium carrots
- 1 pound of sweet potatoes
- 1 celery stalk
- 2 tbsp of extra virgin olive oil
- Chili powder to taste
- 4 cups of vegetable
- ½ pound of kale
- 6 walnuts

Directions:

1. Peel and cut in small cubes the onions, garlic, carrots, sweet potatoes, and celery stalk. Heat the oil in the pan. Add the cubed vegetables and simmer for 3 minutes. Add chili and salt, if needed.

2. Add the stock and let the soup simmer for 20 minutes. In the meantime, wash and destem the kale. Blanch the kale within 1 to 2 minutes in boiling salted water.

3. Heat oil in a pan and add the kale. Fry it for 5 minutes. Cut the walnuts. Puree the soup with a stab mixer, then add yogurt and chili powder to taste. Ladle the soup into 4 bowls and top each bowl with kale and walnuts.

Nutrition: Calories: 213 Fat: 4g Carbs: 44g Protein: 13g

Kale, Apple, and Fennel Soup

Preparation Time: 5 minutes

Cooking Time: 15 minutes

Servings: 3

Ingredients:

- 450g (1lb) kale, chopped
- 200g (7oz) fennel, chopped
- 2 apples, peeled, cored, and chopped
- 2 tablespoons fresh parsley, chopped
- 1 tablespoon olive oil
- Sea salt
- Freshly ground black pepper

Directions:

1. Warm oil in a saucepan, add the kale and fennel, and cook for 5 minutes until the fennel has softened. Stir in the apples and parsley.
2. Cover with hot water, bring it to a boil, and simmer for 10 minutes. Using a hand blender or

food processor, blitz until the soup is smooth. Season with salt and pepper. Serve.

Nutrition: Calories: 100 Fat: 1 g Carbohydrate: 17 g Proteins: 4 g

Lentil Soup

Preparation Time: 5 minutes

Cooking Time: 1 hour and 5 minutes

Servings: 4

Ingredients:

- 175g (6oz) red lentils
- 1 red onion, chopped
- 1 clove of garlic, chopped
- 2 sticks of celery, chopped
- 2 carrots, chopped
- ½ birds-eye chili
- 1 teaspoon ground cumin
- 1 teaspoon ground turmeric
- 1 teaspoon ground coriander (cilantro)
- 1200mls (2 pints) vegetable stock (broth)
- 2 tablespoons olive oil
- Sea salt

- Freshly ground black pepper

Directions:

1. Warm-up oil in a saucepan and add the onion and cook for 5 minutes. Add in the carrots, lentils, celery, chili, coriander (cilantro), cumin, turmeric, and garlic and cook for 5 minutes.

2. Pour in the stock (broth), bring it to the boil, reduce the heat and simmer for 45 minutes. Puree the soup using your hand blender or food processor—season with salt and pepper. Serve.

Nutrition: Calories: 94 Fat: 1g Carbs: 34g Protein: 13g

Spicy Pumpkin Soup

Preparation Time: 17 minutes

Cooking Time: 28 minutes

Servings: 4

Ingredients:

- 150g (5oz) kale
- 1 butternut squash, peeled, de-seeded, and chopped
- 1 red onion, chopped
- 3 bird's-eye chilies, chopped
- 3 cloves of garlic
- 2 teaspoons turmeric
- 1 teaspoon ground ginger
- 600mls (1 pint) vegetable stock (broth)
- 2 tablespoons olive oil

Directions:

1. Warm-up olive oil in a saucepan, add the chopped butternut squash and onion and cook for 6 minutes until softened.

2. Stir in the kale, garlic, chili, turmeric, ginger, and cook for 2 minutes, stirring constantly. Pour in the vegetable stock (broth), bring it to the boil, and cook for 20 minutes.

3. Process until smooth using your food processor or a hand blender. Serve. Enjoy.

Nutrition: Calories: 164 Carbs: 32g Protein: 22g Fat: 3g

French Onion Soup

Preparation Time: 5 minutes

Cooking Time: 55 minutes

Servings: 4

Ingredients:

- 750g (1¾ lbs.) red onions, thinly sliced
- 50g (2oz) Cheddar cheese, grated (shredded)
- 12g (½ oz.) butter
- 2 teaspoons flour
- 2 slices whole meal bread
- 900mls (1½ pints) vegetable stock (broth)
- 1 tablespoon olive oil

Directions:

1. Warm butter and oil in a large pan. Add the onions and gently cook on low heat for 25 minutes, stirring occasionally.

2. Add in the flour and stir well. Pour in the stock (broth) and keep stirring. Boil, reduce the heat, and simmer for 30 minutes.

3. Cut the slices of bread into triangles, sprinkle with cheese and place them under a hot grill (broiler) until the cheese has melted. Serve the soup into bowls and add 2 triangles of cheesy toast on top. Enjoy.

Nutrition: Calories: 92 Fat: 3g Carbs: 511g Protein: 2g

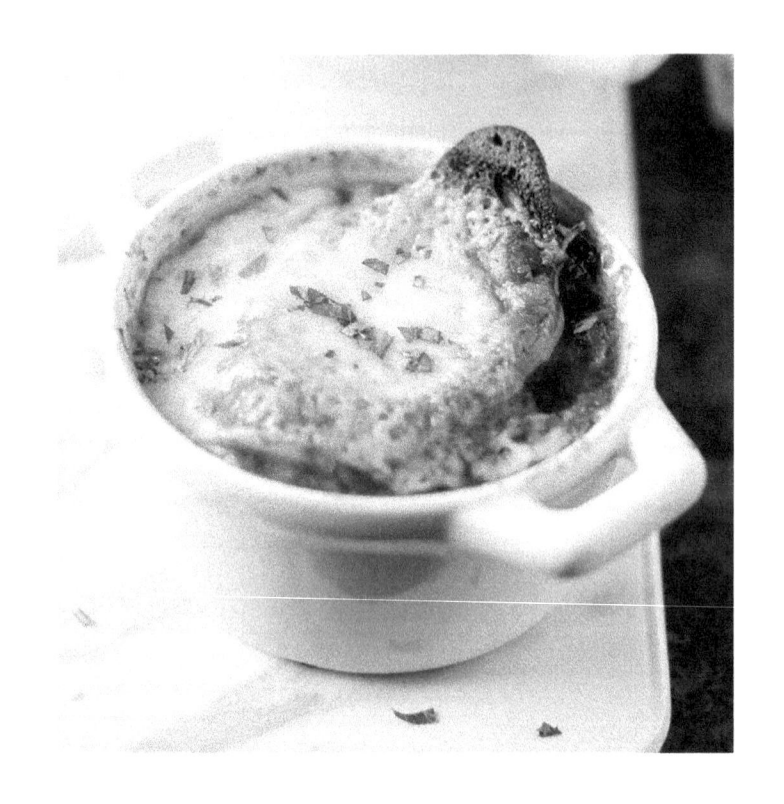

Creamy Broccoli and Kale Soup

Preparation Time: 5 minutes

Cooking Time: 30 minutes

Servings: 4

Ingredients:

- 250g (9oz) broccoli
- 250g (9oz) kale
- 1 potato, peeled and chopped
- 1 red onion, chopped
- 600mls (1 pint) vegetable stock
- 300mls (½ pint) milk
- 1 tablespoon olive oil
- Sea salt
- Freshly ground black pepper

Directions:

1. Warm-up olive oil in a saucepan, add the onion, and cook for 5 minutes. Add in the potato, kale, and broccoli and cook for 5 minutes.

2. Pour in the stock (broth) and milk and simmer for 20 minutes. Using a food processor or hand blender, process the soup until smooth and creamy—season with salt and pepper. Re-heat if necessary and serve.

Nutrition: Calories: 100 Fat: 4g Carbs: 4g Protein: 8g

Creamy Asparagus Soup

Preparation Time: 10 minutes

Cooking Time: 0 minutes

Servings: 2

Ingredients:

- 12 asparagus spears, trimmed
- 1 avocado, pitted and peeled
- A pinch of salt and white pepper
- 1 yellow onion, peeled and chopped
- 3 cups of water

Directions:

1. Add the mushrooms with asparagus, avocado, onion, water, salt, and pepper in your blender. Pulse well, divide into soup bowls, and serve right away. Heat if desired.

Nutrition: Calories: 123.3 Fat: 4.4g Carbs: 16.3g Protein: 31g

Creamy white asparagus soup

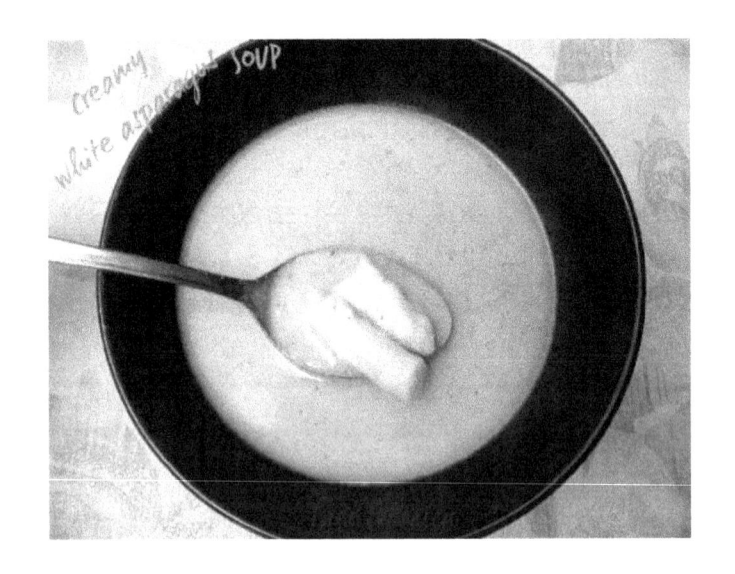

CPSIA information can be obtained
at www.ICGtesting.com
Printed in the USA
BVHW081255250521
608098BV00004B/736